Published By Adam Gilbin

@ Alvin Pinner

Wheat Belly: The Complete Easy and Wheat-free

Recipes to Lose Weight and Feel Good

ISBN 978-1-990666-89-6

I0105876

TABLE OF CONTENTS

Oat & Date Cookies

Ingredients:

- ½ tsp ground cinnamon

- ¼ cup canola oil

- ½ tsp baking powder

- 1 egg

- 3 tbsp hot water

- 1 ½ cups rolled oats

- ¼ cup maple syrup

- ½ tsp vanilla extract

- A pinch of salt

- ¼ tsp baking soda

- 3 oz date paste

- ¾ cup quinoa, cooked

- ¼ cup finely chopped nuts

- ½ cup chopped dried fruit

Directions:

1. Preheat oven to 350F.
2. Cover a baking tray with baking parchment or another appropriate non-stick surface.
3. In a food processor, blend the oats to a rough flour.
4. Pour the oat flour into a mixing bowl and combine it with cinnamon, baking powder, salt and baking soda. Set aside for later.
5. Next, blend together the wet Ingredients: using a food processor.
6. Transfer the wet Ingredients: into the mixing bowl with the dry Ingredients:.
7. Beat until both mixtures are combined and a wet dough is produced.

8. Toss in the dried fruit and stir to ensure an even distribution. Set aside the dough for 15 minutes.

9. Place the dough onto the baking tray in 9 evenly distributed portions, approximately 1 ½ cm high.

10. Bake for 30 minutes, until the cookies are soft.

11. Leave to cook on a rack for at least 10 minutes before serving.

Simple Cherry Dessert

Ingredients:

- 1 cup walnuts, roughly chopped

- 4 tsp fresh lemon juice

- 4 ½ cups red cherries, pitted

- ¼ cup water

- ¼ cup caster sugar

- 7 cups Greek yogurt

- ¼ cup almond syrup

Directions:

1. Combine the wet Ingredients:, except for the yogurt, in a bowl and stir thoroughly.
2. Add the cherries and transfer to a saucepan and bring to the boil.

3. Stir occasionally to ensure the liquid doesn't burn.
4. Transfer the cherry syrup into a container and leave to cool.
5. Serve the cherry syrup and cherries alongside Greek yogurt and a sprinkling of chopped walnuts.

Paleo White Chocolate

Ingredients:

- 1 teaspoon of vanilla powder

- 2 ounces coconut milk powder

- Tiny pinch of salt

- 1 teaspoon cacao nibs (optional for inside your chocolates)

- 1/4 cup of raw cacao butter, melted

- 1 teaspoon maple sugar

Directions:

1. Melt your raw cocoa butter in a glass bowl over a double boiler on your stove set to low (raw cocoa melts at 93 degrees, don't burn it).

2. Once melted, transfer to another bowl and add the remaining Ingredients:.

3. Whisk well ensuring there are no lumps left and everything is incorporated.
4. Transfer to a blender or a food processor and run it to get it as smooth as possible.
5. Pour into your chocolate molds or silicon cups and place in the freezer for at least an hour.
6. Remove and serve or chop them up and add them to chocolate chip cookies or muffins

Paleo Chocolate Chip Pizookie

Ingredients:

- Chips (soy free, dairy free)

- 1 organic cage-free egg

- 1/3 cup raw honey (melted)

- 1/4 cup coconut oil (melted)

- 1/2 teaspoon vanilla Extract

- 2 cups sifted blanched almond flour

- 1/2 teaspoon baking soda

- 1/4 teaspoon sea salt

- 1 cup Enjoy Life Mini Chocolate

Directions:

1. Preheat oven to 350 ˚F.

2. Grease mini 6" cast iron skillets. In a large bowl, mix together the almond flour, baking soda, and salt with a fork.

3. Add the chocolate chips to the dry mixture and combine.

4. In a small separate bowl, mix the wet Ingredients: together, honey, coconut oil, vanilla extract, and egg.

5. You may need to heat the honey and coconut oil in order to liquefy them, remember to heat before you add the egg.

6. Stir the wet Ingredients: into the dry until evenly mixed.

7. Let the dough chill in the fridge for at least 30 minutes.

8. Then fill both skillets evenly with dough.

9. Bake for 30-35 minutes or until a toothpick comes out clean.

10. Garnish with coconut milk ice cream and enjoy!

Talk Of The Town Tofu

Ingredients:

- 1/4 cup skim milk

- 3 tablespoons sesame seeds

- 1 cup firm tofu, chopped into bite size pieces

- 1 tablespoon garlic powder

- Salt to taste

Directions:

1. Preheat the oven to 400 degrees F, spray a baking sheet with no stick spray.
2. Combine the garlic powder and skim milk, and then pour in the tofu.
3. Pick up the pieces of tofu and place them on the baking sheet.

4. Sprinkle with sesame seeds and bake in the oven for 30 minutes, flipping half way through.

5. Season with salt, to taste.

6. This tofu is a perfect garnish or addition to a variety of dishes, or they are perfect to eat as is. High in protein and low calorie, you can't go wrong with tofu!

The Nutty Procession

Ingredients:

- 1/2 cup chocolate chips, melted

- 1/2 cup peanut butter

- 1/2 cup peanuts

- 1/2 cup cashews

Directions:

1. Line a cookie sheet with freezer paper.
2. Melt the chocolate chips on the stove, then transfer to a small mixing bowl, mix in peanut butter immediately.
3. Crush the peanuts and cashews into small pieces, and then add to the peanut butter chocolate. Stir. The batter will be thick.
4. Spread onto the freezer paper, and then place in freezer for 25 minutes.

5. Once frozen, cut into candy bar sized pieces and serve.

6. Guaranteed to give you the energy boost you need, without all of the carbs and calories, make these up on a hot summer's day, and cool down while you slim down.

Breaded Cheese Dunkers And Yogurt Dip

Ingredients:

- 1 egg, beaten

- 1/2 cup plain, low fat yogurt

- 1 tablespoon parsley

- 3 slices potato bread

- 6 strings string cheese

Directions:

1. Finely crumble the bread until it is completely crumbs.
2. Preheat your oven to 350 degrees F, and spray a baking sheet with no stick.
3. Take the cheese sticks, and dip them in the egg, then roll them in the bread crumbs until completely covered.
4. Lie on baking sheet and put in oven for 10 minutes.

5. While the cheese is baking, mix the parsley into the yogurt, stirring until it is creamy, but not too thin.

6. Remove the cheese from the oven, and serve with the dip.

7. This is a light and refreshing, high protein dish that will keep you satisfied.

8. No need to worry about wheat or carbs on this one, it is all about low calories, and high protein. Don't forget it tastes great, too!

Breakfast Biscuits With Egg

Ingredients:

- 4 teaspoons baking powder

- 4 tablespoons cold butter cut it into cubes

- 4 egg whites

- This recipe serves eight people.

- 1 cup almond flour/meal

- 1 cup ground flaxseed

Directions:

1. Preheat your oven to 350F. Line your baking sheet with parchment paper.

2. Mix together in a large sized bowl your almond flour/meal, flaxseed and baking powder. Use your butter cubes until everything is mixed.

3. Beat your egg whites in a medium sized bowl on high until you notice soft peaks forming. Fold your egg whites into your flour and Ingredients: until they are well blended.

4. Spoon this dough into eight round balls on your baking sheet.

5. Flatten until they are about 3/4 inch thick. Bake for 12-15 minutes – less, if they are turning golden brown.

Yummy Miniature Pizzas

Ingredients:

- 1/2 cup ground flaxseed

- 1 teaspoon sea salt

- 2 tablespoons olive oil

- 1 1/2 cups sugar-free marinara or pizza sauce

- 3/4 cup of warm water

- 1 1/4 teaspoons active dry yeast

- 1 cup almond flour/meal

- 1 cup chickpea flour

Toppings are optional:

- Thin sliced, sautéed onion and bell pepper

- Thin sliced, sautéed zucchini and yellow squash

- Grape tomatoes – quartered

- 2 tablespoons fresh, chopped herbs

- 1 cup mozzarella cheese – shredded

- 1 cup ricotta cheese

- 4 oz thin-sliced pepperoni

- 8 oz thin sliced mozzarella cheese – fresh

Directions:

1. Whisk the yeast and water in a small sized bowl until the yeast fully dissolves.
2. Allow this to stand for 10 minutes.
3. Whisk the almond flour/meal, chickpea flour, salt and flaxseed in a medium bowl.

4. Add the yeast and oil mixture and stir together for five minutes, until all of your Ingredients: are distributed evenly and formed into a ball of dough.

5. Cover the dough ball with plastic wrap and allow it to stand in a warm area for one hour.

6. Then divide the ball into six equal pieces.

7. Preheat your oven to 350F. Line two baking sheets with parchment paper.

8. Use a piece of the same type of parchment paper on your work surface.

9. Place one dough piece on parchment paper and top it with a second parchment paper sheet.

10. Flatten it into a four-inch circle with a rolling pin.

11. Place your dough circle on a baking sheet.

12. Remove the top parchment paper carefully.

13. Use your hands or a spoon to form the crust edge.

14. Repeat these steps with the other dough pieces.
15. Bake the dough pieces for 20 minutes, or until they are lightly brown.
16. Then remove them from the oven and top them with 1/4 cup marinara or pizza sauce and your favorite toppings.
17. Bake for 10 more minutes or until they are heated all the way through.

Wheat & Gluten Free Almond Butter Energy Bars Recipe

Ingredients:

- 1 tbsp raw cacao powder

- 2 tbsp cacao nibs

- 3 tbsp chia seeds

- 3 tbsp sunflower or pumpkin seeds

- 225g gluten free oats

- 125g almond butter

- 3 scoops chocolate protein powder (we used Kaizen 100% Whey Isolate in Decadent Chocolate flavour 1 scoop = 1/3 cup = 40g)

- 125ml water

- 1 tsp almond extract

22

Directions:

1. Line a baking tray 17cm square (7" square) with baking paper.
2. Put all the dry ingredients into a food mixer with dough attachment, and mix until well distributed.
3. Add the almond butter and water.
4. It takes a bit of effort to get everything combined.
5. If the mix still looks too dry then add ½ tbsp of water at a time.
6. Do not add too much extra water as the mixture will very quickly turn too soft. Hint: if this does happen simply add more oats until the mixture is fairly stiff again.
7. Spoon the mixture into the prepared pan and spread about equally, press the mixture flat with the back of a spoon. This will compress it into solid bars.

8. Cover and put in the freezer for approximately 30 minutes, remove from freezer and cut into bars.

9. Store in the fridge in an airtight container.

Wheat Free Apricot Flapjack Recipe

Ingredients:

- 90ml rice syrup (substitute: Tate & Lyle golden syrup)

- 400g fresh apricots (dried can be substituted and you will only need 250g, but you should soak them before use)

- 50g pine nuts

- 50g raisins

- 225g gluten free oats

- 75g rice flour

- 150g low fat spread, margarine or butter

- Please note this recipe contains pine nuts

Directions:

1. Preheat oven: 180°C, 350°F, Gas 4
2. Line a shallow baking tray 15cm x 25cm (6" x 10") with baking parchment.
3. Gently melt the fat and the rice syrup together.
4. Stir in the oats, flour, pine nuts and raisins, until well mixed. If the mixture is too wet then add more oats, a tablespoon at a time. However Make sure the mixture does not become dry or it will not stick together when cooked.
5. Remove the stones from the fresh apricots and chop.
6. Tip half of the oat mixture into the baking tray and press down firmly, ensuring the mix is well compacted.

7. Spread the apricots on top, then finish off with the rest of the oat mixture, to make an 'apricot sandwich'. Press down firmly, again ensuring the mix is well compacted, but not squashed if using fresh apricots.

8. Bake in the centre of the oven for 25 minutes.

9. As soon as the flapjacks are removed from the oven, cut into squares then allow to cool completely before removing from tray.

10. If you are using dried apricots you will need to soak them for about 30 minutes in a small amount of orange juice to soften them. You can substitute other dried fruits for the raisins, i.e. dried cranberries or cherries.

Creamy Yogurt Fresh Fruit Salad

Ingredients:

- 1 8-ounce compartment of vanilla or plain yogurt

- 1 teaspoon sugar

- 2 teaspoons lemon juice

- ½ teaspoon vanilla extract

- 2 cups strawberries, sliced

- 2 bananas, sliced

- 2 new peaches, sliced

- 2 cups grapes

- Lime juice

Directions:

1. Mix all the natural product together in a major bowl

2. Mix in around 3 tablespoons of lime juice to keep the natural products from going brown.

3. This likewise assists with supporting the flavor.

4. Mix yogurt, sugar, lemon juice, and vanilla in a little bowl.

5. You have the choice to either serve the yogurt blend as a plunge for the organic products, or blend it right in with the natural product to make a salad.

6. Serve right away

Banana Ice Cream With A Twist

Ingredients:

- 4 bananas that are marginally overripe, cut and frozen

- 2 tablespoons smooth nut butter

- 2 teaspoons cocoa powder

- Optional: milk

Directions:

1. Place frozen banana cuts in a food processor and pulse.
2. You can add milk to assist the bananas with mixing faster.
3. When the bananas begin to appear as though whipped frozen yogurt, you can include the peanut butter and cocoa powder.
4. For a delicate serve frozen yogurt surface, serve it immediately.

5. For a firmer surface, you can pop it in the cooler first.

Baked Yam Sticks

Ingredients:

- ½ teaspoon paprika

- 4 yams

- 1 tablespoon olive oil

Directions:

1. Preheat oven to 400o F. Spray a baking sheet pan with oil.
2. In a large bowl, add oil and pepper. Add the potatoes cut into strips; mix well.
3. Place them on the baking sheet.
4. Bake 40 minutes in oven. Remove when done and enjoy.

Zucchini 'Noodles

Ingredients:

- 1 clove garlic, minced

- salt and pepper to taste

- ¼ cup Parmesan cheese

- 6 zucchini

- 2 teaspoons salt

- 3 tablespoons margarine

Directions:

1. Cut zucchini into thin pasta like strips. Mix with 2 teaspoons salt and place into a colander to drain for 30 minutes.

2. Add water in a pot and bring to boil. Add zucchini; cook one minute.

3. Drain; Rinse immediately with cold water.

4. Heat the margarine on medium-high heat.

5. Add zucchini and garlic; cook and stir until tender, about 5 minutes.
6. Season with salt and pepper. Sprinkle with Parmesan cheese.

Chicken And Avocado Wrap

Ingredients:

- ½cup cheddar cheese

- 1 tbsp. sugar-free salad dressing

- ½cup bean sprouts

- Prepared flaxseed wrap

- 2 cups spinach leaves

- 8 oz. roasted chicken breast (diced)

- ½avocado (pitted and chopped)

Directions:

1. Lay the flaxseed wraps and then lay the diced chicken, avocado, spinach, bean sprouts, and top with cheese.
2. Drizzle with sugar-free salad dressing and then roll.

Baked Pork Patty

Ingredients:

- ½tsp. fennel

- salt and pepper to taste

- 2 tbsp. almond flour

- ½tsp. baking soda

- 2 tbsp. flax flour

- 8 whole eggs

- 3 oz. grated mozzarella.

- ½cup grated cheddar cheese

- 16 oz. ground pork

- 2 tbsp. olive oil

- 1 medium onion (diced)

- 2 celery stalks (chopped)

- 2 clove garlic (minced)

- ½tsp. sage

- 6 eggs (to top the pork patty)

Directions:

1. Preheat oven at 350°F

2. Heat olive oil in pan in medium fire. Saute the onion and celery and then add the ground pork.

3. Season with garlic, sage, fennel, salt and pepper.

4. Add the almond flour, baking soda, flax flour, eggs, and mozzarella.

5. Place the cooked ground pork mixture in a baking dish and top with cheddar cheese.

6. Cook in the oven for 20 mins.

7. Remove from oven and then crack the six eggs on top.

8. Place back in the oven until the eggs are cooked through.

Fettuccine Alfredo Wheat Belly Style

Ingredients:

- ¾ cup of Parmesan cheese (grated)

- ¼ cup of pecorino romano cheese (grated)

- ¼ teaspoon of black pepper (ground)

- A pinch of red pepper (ground)

- 1 tablespoon of parsley (minced)

- 3 packages of shritake fettuccine (drained and rinsed)

- 4 tablespoons of butter

- 1 clove of minced garlic

- ¾ cup of heavy cream

Directions:

1. Prepare a large sized pot with water and bring to boil. Follow cooking Directions: of your fettuccine as directed on the packaging. Drain and set aside.

2. Using the same pot, add butter and sauté butter for about 2 minutes on low heat. Add the pecorino cheese, parmesan cheese, cream, pepper, red pepper and salt.

3. Cook for about 2 minutes or until cooked thoroughly. Add fettuccine and toss lightly to coat evenly.

4. Transfer to plate. Sprinkle some parsley on top. Serve hot and enjoy!

Cream Of Mushroom

Ingredients:

- Sea salt and pepper for tasting

- 3 cups of chicken stock

- 12 oz of canned coconut milk (choose the thicker variety)

- 2 tablespoons of chopped chives

- 2 tablespoons of EVOO (extra virgin olive oil)

- 1 medium sized yellow onion (chopped finely)

- 2 cloves of minced garlic

- 16 oz of mushrooms (you can choose either button mushrooms, cremini or baby bella; finely

chopped)

Directions:

1. Using a large skillet, heat the olive oil over medium to high heat.

2. Sauté the garlic and onions until fragrant and translucent.

3. Add mushrooms and reduce heat. Season to taste and cover until the mushrooms are cooked through and become soft.

4. Add the coconut milk and chicken stock and cover.

5. Simmer for about 3-5 minutes.

6. Once the soup is done, pour over a blender and pulse until it becomes smooth and cream.

7. You can do this in batches if the soup does not fit the blender.

8. Serve on a bowl and top it with chives. Enjoy!

Grilled Peach-Glazed Pork Chops

Ingredients:

- 3 cups of peach (sliced)

- 1 tomato (quartered and seeded)

- 2 tablespoons of cider vinegar

- 1 tablespoon of canola oil

- ½ cup of onion (chopped)

- ½ teaspoon of salt

- ¼ cup of salt

- ¼ cup of brown sugar

- 2 cups of water

- 3 cups of ice cubes

- 2 lbs of pork chops (bone-in)

- 2 teaspoon of ginger (minced)

- 2 tablespoons of honey

- ¼ teaspoon of ground pepper

Directions:

1. Dissolve ¼ cup of sugar and salt using boiling water in a heat resistant bowl. Add ice cubes and cool solution before you add the pork chops. Put inside the refrigerator for about 30 minutes to cool.

2. Meanwhile, using a food processor, add tomato, vinegar and peaches. Puree until it becomes smooth. Set it aside.

3. Sauté onion in a saucepan over medium-high heat. Add ginger and cook for about a minute before adding peach puree. Add salt, pepper and honey to taste. Bring to boil.

4. Put the heat to low and simmer the liquid for about 20 minutes or until liquid becomes reduced in half. Keep it warm.

5. Meanwhile, preheat your grill to low to medium high heat. Get the pork chops and drain liquid.

6. Pat dry the meat using a paper towel. Baste the meat with the pureed peach mixture on each side.

7. Grill the pork for about 4 minutes on both sides.

8. Brush them with the pureed peach every now and then.

9. Transfer to a plate and cover it with aluminum foil to rest the meat for about 5 minutes.

10. Serve with a vegetable side dish and add a spoon of peach glaze on the side. Enjoy!

Avocado Stuffed With Spicy Salsa

Ingredients:

- Cayenne pepper (¼ teaspoon)

- Red onion (1/2, finely chopped)

- Lime (1 piece)

- Sea salt (¼ teaspoon)

- Fresh cilantro (3 tablespoons, finely chopped)

- Avocados (4 medium-size pieces, halved and pitted)

- Tomato (1 medium-size piece, finely chopped)

- Poblano pepper (1 piece, finely chopped)

Directions:

1. Get a medium bowl and add in onion, tomato, poblano pepper, cayenne pepper, salt, and cilantro. Mix the Ingredients: well.

2. Get a spoonful of the mixture and place it into each avocado half.

3. Drizzle some fresh lime juice over each avocado half and serve.

Roasted Portobello Mushroom

Ingredients:

- 3 Large Sun-Dried Tomatoes

- Sea Salt to taste

- Olive Oil (or spray)

- 4 to 6 Anchovies (or sardines), chopped (optional)

- 4 large Portobello mushroom-Caps

- 1 Medium Lemon, juiced

- 1 Bunch of Fresh Parsley, diced

- 2 Cloves of Garlic, minced

Directions:

1. Roast the mushrooms in the oven at 400 F for 25 to 30 minutes. Make sure to pull the stalks out.

2. While the mushrooms are cooking, combine all the other Ingredients: in a small bowl and mix.

3. Once the mushrooms are done, top all caps with the sauce and serve!

Strawberry Sesame Spinach Salad

Ingredients:

- 1 teaspoon raw honey

- Pinch dry mustard powder

- Salt and pepper to taste

- 2 tablespoons toasted sesame seeds

- 6 to 8 cups fresh chopped spinach

- 1 ½ cups fresh chopped strawberries

- 3 tablespoons extra-virgin olive oil

- 1 tablespoon balsamic vinegar

Directions:

1. Chop the spinach and divide it among four salad plates.

2. Top each salad with chopped strawberries.

3. Whisk together the remaining Ingredients: aside from the sesame seeds.

4. Drizzle the dressing over the salads and sprinkle with sesame seeds to serve.

Curried Carrot Soup

Ingredients:

- 8 large carrots, peeled and chopped

- 2 large stalks celery, sliced

- ½ tablespoon curry powder

- 6 cups chicken broth

- 2 tablespoons olive oil

- 1 large yellow onion, chopped

- Salt and pepper to taste

Directions:

1. Heat the oil in a stockpot over medium heat.
2. Add the onion, carrots and celery then cook for 10 minutes, stirring occasionally.

3. Stir in the chicken broth and curry powder then bring to a boil.

4. Reduce heat and simmer for 10 minutes until the carrots are tender.

5. Remove from heat and puree the soup using an immersion blender.

6. Season the soup with salt and pepper to taste then serve hot.

Basic Wheat Free Bread

Ingredients:

- 1 teaspoon cinnamon (optional)

- ¼ teaspoon ocean salt

- 5 eggs, differentiated

- ¼ cup butter, liquefied

- 1 tablespoon buttermilk

- 1 tablespoon xylitol or 4 drops fluid stevia or to coveted sweetness

- 1¼ cups whitened almond flour

- ¼ cup + 2 tablespoons garbanzo bean (chickpea) flour

- ¼ cup ground brilliant flaxseeds

- 1½ teaspoons baking soda

Directions:

1. Preheat the oven to 350°F.

2. Oil a 8½" × 4½" pan. In a sustenance processor, consolidate the almond flour, garbanzo bean flour, flaxseeds, preparing pop, cinnamon (if utilizing), and salt.

3. Beat until very much mixed. Include the egg yolks, butter, buttermilk, and Xylitol or stevia and heartbeat just until mixed.

4. In an expansive bowl and utilizing an electric blender on high, beat the egg whites until the delicate tops structure.

5. Fill the flour mixture and heartbeat until the egg whites are equitably dispersed, at the same time, don't run the machine at a steady speed.

6. Spread into the pan and prepare for 40 minutes, or until a wooden pick embedded in the middle comes out clean.

7. Cool in the pan for 10 minutes.

Wheat Free Basic Focaccia

Ingredients:

Flavoured oil

- 2 large garlic cloves, minced

- 1–2 tablespoons minced fresh herbs (such as basil or rosemary)

- Add 3 tablespoons of olive oil

- ½ teaspoon fine sea salt

Dough

- ½ cup ground golden flaxseeds

- 2 teaspoons baking powder

- ½ teaspoon fine sea salt

- 1 cup buttermilk

- 1 teaspoon instant (rapid rise) yeast (optional)

- 2 cups almond meal/flour

- 1 cup garbanzo bean (chickpea) flour

- 4 egg whites

Directions:

1. In a small saucepan over low heat, combine the oil, salt, and garlic and simmer for 10 minutes.
2. Remove the saucepan from the heat.
3. Apply a delicate herb, such as basil, add it to the oil after you swallow the oil from the groove.
4. If using a hardier herb, such as rosemary, allow it to simmer for the full 10 minutes. Set aside for later use. (Alternatively, you can go over this step and brush the focaccia with

plain olive oil, then sprinkle your favourite seasonings on top.)

5. Preheat the oven to 400°F. Grease a 13" × 9" baking sheet with half of the oil, seam it with

6. Parchment paper, and then generously brush the paper with the reserved oil.

7. In a large bowl, blend the almond meal/flour, garbanzo bean flour, flax seeds, baking powder, and salt.

8. Stir or whisk to blend and split up the flour.

9. In a small bowl or glass measure, whisk the buttermilk and yeast, if using, until the yeast dissolves.

10. Set aside for later use. In a separate bowl, whip the egg whites with mixer until stiff peaks form.

11. Add the yeast mix to the flour mixture and shake until a rough dough ball forms.

12. Gently fold in the egg whites until they're fairly well integrated.

13. The dough will not become totally smooth, and the whites will still be slightly frothy.

14. Spread the dough in the pan with a spatula or spoon.

15. Lightly coat your fingertips with cooking spray or dip them into the reserved oil and dimple the top of the bread.

16. Pour the remaining oil mixture over the upper side of the dough, making certain it is totally covered. (Oil will pool in the dimples.)

17. Bake for 20 minutes or until golden and slightly spongy in the centre.

18. With a pizza cutter or knife, cut into the desired size and number of flat breads. Serve while still slightly warm.

Spinach Salad

Ingredients:

- 1 c. walnuts

- ¼ c. currants

- 2 tbsp. balsamic vinegar

- 2 tbsp. olive oil

- 5 cups baby spinach

- 1 apple, halved

Directions:

1. Toast the walnuts over low heat in an iron skillet for approximately 10 minutes or until brown.
2. Place the spinach, currants, and apple sticks into a bowl.
3. Combine the spinach salad with the walnuts and toss.

4. Drizzle with the vinegar and olive oil before serving.

Orange Arugula Salad

Ingredients:

- 3 tbsp. Olive oil

- 1 tbsp. Balsamic vinegar

- 2 oranges, segmented

- 4 c. Arugula

- Salt

Directions:

1. Combine the oranges and arugula in the salad bowl.
2. Drizzle the oil and vinegar with a dash of salt.
3. Toss them together then serve.

Simple Avocado Smoothie

Ingredients:

- 1 tbsp caster sugar

- 1 tbsp fresh basil, chopped

- 1 ripe avocado, halved, pitted &
  fleshed

- 1 ¼ cups milk

- 2 tbsp fresh lime juice

Directions:

1. Add all Ingredients: to a food processor and
   process until smooth.
2. Separate into two glasses, sprinkle with basil
   and serve.
3. You may also wish to add a little ice before
   serving.

Nutty Sweets

Ingredients:

- ½ cup sugar

- 2 egg whites

- ½ tsp sunflower oil

- 1 cup roasted almonds

- 1 cup walnuts

Directions:

1. Preheat oven to 300F.
2. Using low-calorie cooking spray, grease an 8 square inch baking dish.
3. In a food processor, pulse the nuts until a flour is produced.
4. Transfer to a mixing bowl and add the sugar, egg whites. Beat until one mixture is produced.

5. Transfer the sweet mixture onto a baking tray, ensuring an even layer.

6. Cook for 1 hour.

7. Remove the baking tray from the oven and leave to cool for at least 15 minutes.

8. Slice the sweet slab into 16 even pieces.

Almond Granita

Ingredients:

- ½ cup caster sugar

- ¼ cup almond paste

- 1 tsp almond extract

- 1 ¼ cups whole milk

- ½ cup roasted almonds

- 1 ¼ cups water

Directions:

1. In a food processor, blend all Ingredients: until a smooth liquid is produced. Strain the liquid over a fine-sieve, discarding any solids caught.

2. Pour the almond liquid into a 9*9*2 baking tray and freeze for at least 1 hour.

3. Break the frozen almond liquid into flakes.
    Serve immediately.

Blueberry Mango Muffins

Ingredients:

- 1/4 teaspoon salt

- 1/4 teaspoon vanilla

- 1/4 teaspoon baking powder

- 1/4 cup coconut flour

- 1/2 cup diced mango

- 1/2 cup blueberries

- 3 eggs

- 3 tablespoon honey

- 2 tablespoon coconut oil, melted

- 2 tablespoon coconut milk

Directions:

1. Preheat oven to 400°F.

2. Mix together your eggs, honey, coconut oil, coconut milk, salt and vanilla.
3. Sift together your baking powder and coconut flour and then combine with your wet Ingredients:.
4. Mix your batter well and then fold in your diced mango and blueberries.
5. If not, divide your batter into 9 muffin tins and bake for 20 minutes or until done.

Dark Chocolate Fudge Pops

Ingredients:

- 1½ teaspoons unflavored gelatin

- 1 teaspoon vanilla extract

- 2 ounces unsweetened chocolate, roughly chopped

- 1¼ cups coconut milk

- 2 egg yolks

- ½ cup maple syrup or honey

- Dash of sea salt

Directions:

1. Soften the gelatin by placing it in a small bowl with the vanilla extract.

2. Warm the coconut milk over medium-high heat for 6-7 minutes, being careful not to let it

boil. Whisk the egg yolks, maple syrup, and salt in a small bowl.

3. Slowly pour the hot coconut milk into the egg mixture, whisking continuously to temper the eggs.

4. Pour the entire liquid mixture back into the pan, and continue cooking over medium high heat for 6-8 minutes while stirring constantly.

5. You don't want this mixture to boil and it should be thick enough to coat the back of a spoon.

6. Pour the softened gelatin and vanilla into the pan and whisk vigorously until the gelatin has completely dissolved, about 2 minutes.

7. Remove from heat, and pour the mixture into a glass bowl. *If you notice a few small lumps, pass it through a mesh strainer prior to pouring it into the bowl.

8. Stir in the chopped chocolate until it is incorporated and smooth, then let the

pudding cool for 20 minutes at room temperature.

9. Pour the pudding into popsicle molds and freeze for at least 6 hours until solid.

Sweet Spinach Pie With Basic Paleo Almond Crust

Ingredients:

For the pie crust:

- 1 tablespoon coconut oil

- 1 egg

- 1 cup ground almonds (almond flour)

- 1 tablespoon coconut flour

- Pinch of sea salt

For the spinach filling:

- 1 cup ground almonds (almond flour)

- 2 tablespoons coconut flour

- 1 cup coconut sugar

- 1 teaspoon rosewater

- 300g fresh spinach leaves (1 cup cooked)

- 4 eggs, separated

- Pinch of sea salt

Directions:

For the crust:

1. In a mixing bowl, knead all the Ingredients: together until a dough is formed.

2. With your hands, press the dough into a pie plate, bottom and sides (I used a 6-inch round plate). Set aside.

For the spinach filling:

3. In a medium-sized pot, place the spinach and about 1 cup of water.

4. At medium heat, bring to a boil, and cook about 5 minutes.

5. Reduce the heat to low and cook an additional 5 minutes.
6. Turn heat off and allow to cool in the pot with water.
7. Once the spinach is cool, drain into a colander and press the spinach to remove all of the water.
8. I pressed it with the back of a spoon. Put the spinach, egg yolks, rosewater and sea salt into a food processor. Pulse until a puree is formed, about 1 minute.
9. Add the almond four, coconut flour and sugar and pulse again until everything is well incorporated.
10. Pour the dough into a mixing bowl. Beat the egg whites until stiff peaks form.
11. Fold the egg whites into the spinach mixture.
12. Mix well until no white is visible.
13. Pour the spinach filling into the pie crust.

14. Bake at 180°C (350°F) for 35-45 minutes, or until an inserted toothpick comes out dry.

Peanut Butter Power Drink

Ingredients:

- 1 cup skim milk

- 1 tablespoon honey

- 1/4 cup peanut butter

- 1/2 cup vanilla yogurt

Directions:

1. Toss everything into a blender and blend on high until it is completely liquid. Add more milk for a thinner consistency.

2. This is one of the fastest and easiest recipes that you can imagine.

3. Taking only minutes to make, you will burn more calories in clean up than this dish provides.

Cheddar Scrambled Egg Mugs

Ingredients:

- Salt and pepper to taste

- 1/4 cup skim milk

- 1 egg

- 1/4 cup shredded cheese

Directions:

1. Place egg and milk in a coffee mug and whip together.
2. Place in the microwave, and microwave on high for 1 minute.
3. Carefully remove and add cheese, then microwave for an additional 30 seconds.
4. This is a super easy and fast snack that could even work for a busy morning breakfast.
5. Conveniently contained in a coffee mug, this scrambled egg delight is just what you need to

curb the hunger, and still avoid those pesky carbs.

6. Go ahead, grab a mug and try it for yourself.

Full Green Bean Casserole

Ingredients:

- 16 ounces thawed green beans, French-cut

- 8 ounces cubed cream cheese

- 3 tablespoons Parmesan cheese, grated

- 1 cup chicken broth

- 1/8 teaspoon red pepper, ground

- 4 tablespoons coconut oil or butter, divided

- 1/4 cup ground flaxseed

- 1 large onion, yellow – chopped

- 1 large onion, yellow – cut into rings

- 4 ounces sliced button mushrooms

Directions:

1. Preheat oven to 350F. Grease a 2-quart baking dish.
2. Over medium heat in a large skillet, heat 2 of 4 tablespoons of oil or butter.
3. Add your onion rings and cook them.
4. Stir occasionally as they cook for about 10 minutes, or until they are lightly browned.
5. Place flaxseeds on a plate. Add your browned onion rings and coat with flaxseed. Set them to the side.
6. Using the same skillet on medium-high heat, add the other 2 tablespoons of oil or butter and heat.
7. Cook mushrooms and chopped onion for eight minutes, until they absorb most of the liquid.
8. Add broth and green beans and heat to simmer.
9. Stir in cream cheese until it melts.

10. Stir in red pepper and Parmesan cheese.

11. Pour mixture into your baking dish and arrange onion rings on top.

12. Bake the casserole for about 25 minutes, until it is bubbling and hot.

Onion Rings For A Green Bean Casserole

Ingredients:

- 1/2 cup almond meal

- 1 cup ground flaxseed

- 2 sweet onions, large in size, separated in rings after being cut into 1/2 inch thick slices

- 3/4 cup divided coconut flour

- 1/2 teaspoon smoked paprika

- 1 egg

- 1 tablespoon melted olive or coconut oil

Directions:

1. Preheat your oven to 450F. Spray cooking spray to coat two baking sheets.

2. Combine one quarter cup of paprika and coconut flour in a small bowl.

3. Using another bowl, beat the oil and egg until they are blended.

4. Use a large plate to combine the almond meal, 1/2 cup of coconut flour and the flaxseed.

5. Drench onion rings in the paprika-coconut flour mixture.

6. Shake off any extra mixture gently. Dip the rings into the egg mixture, and allow the excess to drip off.

7. Coat with the flaxseed mixture. Place onion rings on baking sheets and coat lightly with the cooking spray.

8. Bake onion rings for 12 minutes or until browned. Turn them once while baking.

Wheat & Gluten Free Apple Berry Oat Bars Recipe

Ingredients:

- 375ml unsweetened apple purée

- 60g dried cranberries (I used fruit apple sweetened ones)

- 45g unsweetened shredded coconut

- 30g chopped walnuts

- 2 tsp chia seeds

- 250g gluten free oats (regular, not quick or flake)

- 1 large organic apples, cored and finely chopped (leave the skin on)

- 150g fresh blueberries

Directions:

1. Preheat oven: 180°C, 350°F, Gas 4

2. Line a baking pan 23cm square (9" square) with baking paper.

3. Put all the ingredients, except the blueberries, in a large bowl and mix together until they are well combined.

4. Add the blueberries and gently fold them into the mixture, trying not to burst them.

5. Tip into the baking pan and spread equally, press down firmly to consolidate.

6. Bake for 30 minutes, remove from oven and immediately lift the apple berry oat bars from the pan still in the baking paper, leave to cool on a wire rack.

7. When cool, cut into 8 large bars or 16 smaller ones.

8. Store in the fridge in an airtight container.

Wheat Free Autumn Apple Cake Recipe

Ingredients:

- 3⁄4 tsp baking powder

- 1⁄2 tsp bicarbonate of soda

- 1⁄2 tsp xanthan gum

- 1 tsp mixed spice (substitute: cinnamon)

- pinch salt

- 25g butter, margarine, or low fat spread, melted

- 100g greek yogurt or set natural yogurt

- 60ml milk (substitute: almond, rice, soy etc)

- 2 tbsp honey (substitute: agave syrup)

- 1 small egg, beaten

- 110g all purpose wheat free flour (we used Stamp Collection)

- 25g gluten free oats

- 25g unrefined sugar

- 25g raisins

- 25g hazelnuts, whole

- 25g almonds, 50% chopped, 50% left whole

- 1 apple, cored and chopped roughly

- 1 1/2 tsp gluten free oats (to sprinkle on top of cake)

- Please note this recipe contains nuts

Directions:

1. Preheat oven: 200°C, 400°F, Gas 6
2. Line a 16 cm (6 1/2") cake tin with baking parchment.
3. In a large mixing bowl place the flour, oats, sugar, raisins, half the hazelnuts, the chopped almonds, apple, baking powder, bicarbonate of soda, xanthan gum, mixed spice and salt. Stir to mix.
4. In a separate bowl mix together the melted butter, egg, milk, honey and yogurt.
5. Then pour onto the dry ingredients.
6. Gently mix the wet and dry ingredients together, leaving the mix lumpy but with no dry patches.
7. Drop the mixture into the cake tin in spoonfuls, leaving it very uneven on the surface.

8. (The mix will spread to fill the gaps during cooking).

9. Scatter the remaining hazelnuts and whole almonds over the top, and then sprinkle 1½ tsp of oats on the top.

10. Cook on the centre shelf of the oven for 45 minutes.

11. The cake should be covered loosely with foil after the first 25 minutes to stop the nuts burning.

12. To check whether the cake is cooked completely, insert a toothpick into the centre of the cake, if it comes out clean the cake is cooked.

13. Leave the cake to cool in its tin for about 15 minutes before turning out onto a wire rack, removing the baking parchment and leaving to cool completely.

14. This cake can be eaten slightly warm if desired, however it will be fairly fragile until it has cooled and set.

15. Serve with a generous helping of custard, creme fraiche, or cream as a dessert.

Wheat & Gluten Free Banana Oat Energy Bars

Recipe

Ingredients:

- 60g dried cranberries (I use apple juice sweetened ones)

- 45g unsweetened shredded coconut

- 30g chopped walnuts

- 1 tsp chia seeds

- 250g gluten free oats (regular, not quick or flake)

- 2 large ripe bananas, mashed

- 110g apple peach purée (I used an unsweetened fruit snack cup [check it's vegan if required], you can also make your own fruit

purée)

Directions:

1. Preheat oven: 180°C, 350°F, Gas 4

2. Line a baking pan 23cm square (9" square) with baking paper.

3. Put all the Ingredients: in a large bowl and mix together until they are well combined.

4. Tip into the baking pan and spread equally, press down to consolidate.

5. Bake for 30 minutes, remove from oven and immediately lift the banana oat bars from the pan still in the baking paper, leave to cool on a wire rack.

6. When cool, cut into 8 large bars or 12-16 smaller ones.

7. Store in the fridge in an airtight container.

Dreamy Walnut Cake

Ingredients:

- ¼ teaspoon salt

- 4 egg whites

- 4 egg yolks

- ½ cup dark walnuts

- 1 ½ cups English walnuts

- 1 cup sugar (separated into segments of two ¼ cups and ½ cup)

- 2 ounces butter

Directions:

1. Toast the pecans first, and afterward let them cool.

2. Grind them finely along with ¼ cup of sugar.

3. In a little pot, cream the spread in addition to a half cup of sugar.

4. The combination needs to become feathery and light.

5. Add the yolks into the blend each in turn.

6. Scratch the bowl, particularly the sides, and afterward beat subsequent to adding one yolk.

7. Fold in the pecans into the egg and margarine combination. Set aside.

8. In an oil free bowl, whisk the egg whites and gradually include the last ¼ cup of sugar.

9. You will see the arrangement of solid pinnacles.

10. Delicately overlay in this blend into the spread combination.

11. Overlay in just a little at a time until everything has been completely and equitably mixed.

12. Pour the substance into a little Bundt or portion pan. Bake at 350 degrees

Rosemary And Sea Salt Flax Crackers

Ingredients:

- ½ cup ground Romano or parmesan cheese

- Kosher or ocean salt for sprinkling

- 1 teaspoon new rosemary, minced

- 1 cup processed or ground flax seeds

- 2 eggs

Directions:

1. Preheat the stove to 350 degrees Fahrenheit. Utilizing a nonstick splash, shower 1-2 treat sheets.
2. Add the fixings as a whole, with the exception of the salt, in a medium bowl.

3. Mix until all that has been completely consolidated. Allow the blend to sit for around 5 minutes.

4. Using nonstick splash, shower an enormous cutting board or a perfect ledge. For ought to likewise splash your rolling pin.

5. Form the batter into a ball shape and set it on the lubed counter.
   Roll it out as dainty as you need. The most slender ones are the best.

6. Using a treat or bread roll shaper, cut a matrix of 1 inch squares on the smoothed dough.
   Using a pie waiter or little spatula, move the singular squares on the treat sheets.

7. Re-roll the extra mixture and cutting everything until all of the batter is gone.
   Sprinkle the top with salt.

8. Bake the wafers for 10 minutes; eliminate from the stove, flip, and afterward prepare 3 minutes.

9. If you wish your wafers to be exceptionally fresh, take a stab at switching off the broiler and afterward set the saltines back inside after they have as of now chilled off a bit, however are still warm to contact.

10. You can leave them inside for about an hour and they will just become dryer and crispier.

11. You can serve this along with a plunge or cheese.

Chocolate Mousse Shots

Ingredients:

- 1 would coconut be able to drain (full-fat or you can likewise utilize coconut cream)

- ¼ cup in addition to 1 tablespoon cocoa or cacao powder

- ½ teaspoon unadulterated vanilla extract

- Sweetener (you can utilize powdered sugar or stevia)

Directions:

1. Open the coconut milk and leave it revealed in the cooler without a cover for the time being.

2. This is just material in the event that the milk isn't quite so thick as mousse.

3. Recollect not to shake the can before you open it.
4. Once the milk has thickened, move it into a bowl and blend in your vanilla, sugar, and cocoa.
5. You can do this utilizing a fork or with mixers.
6. Pipe the mousse into adorable little compartments and store them in the cooler to make them even thicker.

Roasted Brussels Sprouts

Ingredients:

- 1 ½ lb. Brussels sprouts

- 3 tablespoons olive oil

- Salt and pepper to taste

Directions:

1. Preheat oven to 400o F.
2. Cut ends of the Brussels sprouts and outer yellow leaves.
3. Mix in a bowl with olive oil, salt and pepper.
4. Transfer them on a tray and bake for 35-40 minutes, until crisp.
5. Shake the pan often so Brussels sprouts brown evenly.
6. Sprinkle kosher salt, if you like, and serve hot.

Sautéed Apples

Ingredients:

- ½ cup water

- ½ cup brown sugar

- 2 tsp. cornstarch

- 1/4 cup melted butter

- 4 apples

Directions:

1. Cut apples to small pieces. In a skillet, add butter on medium heat; Add apples and cook until soft, about 5 minutes.

2. In a separate bowl add cornstarch and water and mix well.

3. Add this mixture to skillet. Then add brown sugar. Boil for 2 minutes, stirring well.

4. Take skillet out of heat and serve in a bowl with sprinkle of cinnamon.

Coconut Macaroons

Ingredients:

- 1 tablespoon cornstarch

- ¼ teaspoon almond extract

- 1 ½ cups canned cherries

- 2 ½ cups shredded coconut

- 1 cup white sugar

- 6 egg whites

Directions:

1. Preheat oven to 350o F. Line two baking sheets with parchment paper.
2. In a small bowl, add sugar and cornstarch.
3. In a large metal bowl, combine egg whites and almond extract. Place the bowl over a pan of boiling water and heat. Add sugar to the mix. Beat until thick with an electric mixer, about

15 minutes. Stir in coconut. Remove from heat and let cool for 5 minutes.

4. Pour in a piping bag with a tip. Press dough 1 ½ inches apart on baking sheets. Place half a cherry on top of each cookie.

5. Bake for 18-20 minutes or lightly browned up. Cool on baking sheets.

Homemade Chicken Sausage

Ingredients:

- 2 tsp. Almond oil

- 1 onion (diced)

- 1 tbsp. Fresh sage (chopped)

- 1 tbsp. Light brown sugar

- ½ tbsp fennel seed (chopped)

- 16 oz. Ground chicken

- 1 pc. Medium-sized apple (peeled, diced)

- Salt and pepper to taste

Directions:

1. Place a large non-stick pan over medium fire.
2. Drizzle olive oil and sauté the onion.

3. Cook for two minutes, or until the onions soften.

4. Add the apples in the pan and stir for two minutes.

5. Transfer the cooked onions and apples in a bowl and set aside.

6. Add the chicken, sugar, fennel, fresh sage, in the cooked apples and season with salt and pepper.

7. Combine all the Ingredients: well.

8. Coat the same pan with a cooking spray and place over medium fire.

9. Scoop 1/3 cup of the chicken mixture into the pan and flatten into a 3" patty.

10. Cook until the sausages are browned.

Stuffed Turkey Rolls

Ingredients:

- 6 pcs. Basil leaves

- ¼cup sundried tomatoes (slice thinly)

- Olive oil

- Salt and pepper to tast

- 6 pcs. Turkey fillet (thin slices)

- 6 pcs. Mozzarella string cheese (cut into two)

Directions:

1. Preheat oven at 350˚F.
2. Lay the turkey slices on a baking sheet lined with aluminum foil, place two cheese sticks on one turkey slice, top with dried tomato and

one basil leaf and do the same with the remaining fillets.

3. Roll the turkey tightly (you can use toothpicks to lock the rolls)

4. Drizzle the fillets with olive oil and season with salt and pepper.

5. Cook in the oven for 30 mins.

Spiced Grileld Shrimp And Fruity Salsa

Ingredients:

- 32 oz large shrimp

- 1 onion (cut into ¼")

- 2 tbsp. olive oil

Salsa

- 1 tbsp. fresh cilantro (chopped)

- 1 tsp. sugar

- ¼ tsp. salt

- ½ avocado (pitted and chopped)

- 1 pc. mango (peeled and chopped)

- ½ cup bell pepper (chopped)

- 1 tbsp. freshly squeezed lemon juice

Rub

- 2 tbsp. all spice

- 1 tsp. nutmeg (ground)

- 1 tsp. cinnamon powder

- 1 tsp. cayenne pepper

- 1/3 cup paprika

- 4 tbsp. sugar

- 1 tbsp. thyme

- Salt and pepper to taste

Directions:

1. Mix all the Ingredients: for the rub and place in a clean container.
2. Combine all the Ingredients: of the salsa in a bowl and set aside or refrigerate.

3. Peel the shrimps (retain the tail) and remove the veins.
4. Pleace the peeled shrimps in a bowl and then drizzle with oil and sprinkle with the rub and then toss. Make sure that the shrimps are well-coated.
5. Grill the shrimps until they turn pink.
6. Chop the onions and add to the salsa mixture.
7. Serve the grilled shrimps with salsa on the side.

Smoked Trout With Fritters

Ingredients:

- 1 teaspoon of Himalayan sea salt

- 1 tablespoon of coconut oil

- ¾ cup of buckwheat flour

- 200 grams of smoked salmon or trout

- 1 teaspoon of baking powder (gluten free)

- Black pepper

- 2/3 cup of almond milk (unsweetened)

- Zest of 1 lemon

- 2 tablespoons of dill (add more for garnish)

- 1 egg (free-range)

Directions:

1. Whisk egg with pepper and milk.

2. In a separate bowl, sift baking powder, flour and salt.

3. Slowly pour whisked egg to the dry Ingredients:. Stir well until combined completely.

4. Fold in a tablespoon of zest plus the dill.

5. Refrigerate the mixture for about 15 minutes.

6. Once done, heat coconut oil in a large sized frying pan over medium heat. Scoop a tablespoon of the fritter mixture in the pan. Cook for about 1-2 minutes or until the bottom is already brown.

7. Turn on the other side and cook for another 30 seconds to a minute until the fritters are completely cooked.

8. Repeat Directions: on the rest of the mixture. Add more coconut oil if it's needed.

9. Place on a plate and top with the smoked salmon. Squeeze some fresh lemon juice and top with dill.

10. Serve and enjoy!

Scallop Salad

Ingredients:

- 1 tablespoon of sesame oil (do not use the toasted variety)

- A bunch of watercress (washed, pulled)

- 1 packet of sunflower sprouts

- Sea salt

- Black pepper

- EVOO (extra virgin olive oil)

- 3 handfuls of broad beans

- A handful of sugar snap peas (remove the strings)

- 20 pieces of scallops

- Zest of a lemon

- 1 teaspoon of white wine vinegar (fermented naturally)

Directions:

1. Using a large pot, add salt and water. Bring to boil. Blanche quickly the sugar snap peas and transfer immediately to an ice water bath to stop the cooking process and keep it crunchy.

2. Do the same process with the broad beans. Once done, peel the beans and take off the bright green beans inside and set aside together with the sugar snaps. Discard their skin.

3. Meanwhile, toss scallops with sesame oil. Heat a heavy pan over high heat. Sear scallops for about 30 seconds on each side and transfer to a plate and let cool.

4. Toss together sunflower sprouts and watercress in a bowl. Add the beans, scallops and sugar snaps. Season to taste.

5. Plate the salad and drizzle some EVOO. Add some lemon zest and vinegar.
6. Serve and enjoy!

Tomatillo Gazpacho With Shrimp

Ingredients:

- 1 avocado (pitted, peeled and chopped roughly)

- 1 lb of tomatillos (remove the husks and chopped)

- 1 chopped green bell pepper

- 1 jalapeno pepper (chopped and seeded)

- 1 canned veggie or chicken broth

- 2 tablespoons of EVOO (extra virgin olive oil)

- 3 cloves of chopped garlic

- 1 cucumber (chopped roughly and seeded)

- 1 teaspoon of sugar

- ¼ teaspoon of salt

- 1 cup of shrimp (peeled, cooked and chopped)

- ¼ cup of green olives (diced)

- 2 scallions (diagonally sliced)

Directions:

1. Sauté garlic in a tablespoon of olive oil over medium heat.

2. Meanwhile puree half of cucumber, tomatillos, half avocado, jalapeno and bell pepper using a processor or blender until it becomes smooth.

3. Transfer in a large sized bowl and add sugar, salt and broth. This is now your gazpacho.

4. Combine all the remaining cucumber and avocado, olives, scallions and shrimp using another bowl.

5. Drizzle with oil and toss lightly.

6. Plate gazpachos in a bowl and top them with the shrimp mixture.

7. Serve and enjoy!

Mini Bacon And Broccoli Frittatas

Ingredients:

- 6 Whole Eggs

- 4 Egg Whites

- 2 tbsp. Full-fat Coconut Milk

- Extra Virgin Olive Oil

- Sea Salt and Freshly Ground Black Pepper (to taste)

- 1 cup of Organic Bacon, cooked and cut into cubes

- 1 cup of Broccoli, chopped into small pieces

- 1 Onion, minced

Directions:

1. Preheat the oven to 375 F.

2. Use a small amount of olive oil to grease the muffin tray.

3. Put an equal amount of the bacon, broccoli, and onion into the greased muffin cups. Fill it up to about 60%, leaving space for the egg mixture in the next step.

4. In a bowl, whisk together the egg whites, eggs, coconut milk, and salt and pepper to taste.

5. Pour the egg mixture into each muffin cup. Fill the cups almost to the top, but not completely.

6. Put the muffin tray into the oven and cook for about 20 to 22 minutes or until it turns golden brown.

7. Carefully remove the mini frittatas from the tray and serve.

Spanish Meatball And Butter Bean Stew

Ingredients:

- Garlic cloves (3 pieces, crushed)

- Sweet smoked paprika (1 tablespoon)

- Chopped tomatoes (2 x 400g cans)

- Butter beans (400g can, drained)

- Sweetener equivalent to 2 teaspoons sugar

- Parsley (chopped)

- Lean pork (350g, minced)

- Olive oil (2 teaspoon)

- Red onion (1 large piece, chopped)

- Pepper (any color, 2 , sliced)

- Salt and pepper for seasoning

Directions:

1. Season the pork with salt and pepper and shape the pork into small meatballs.

2. Get a large pan and heat the oil.

3. Add the meatballs and cook for 5 minutes.

4. Next, add the onion and pepper to the same pan and cook for another 5 minutes. Stir every now and then.

5. Add the garlic and paprika. Mix well and cook for another minute.

6. Then add the tomatoes and cover the pan with a lid. Let it simmer for 10 minutes.

7. Add the beans, sugar, and seasoning. Then simmer for a further 10 minutes.

8. Finally, place the meatballs with the tomato sauce onto a plate, add some fresh parsley and serve.

Smoked Haddock

Ingredients:

- Carrot (1 piece, finely chopped)

- Dill (2 tbsp., chopped)

- Celery stick (1 piece, finely chopped)

- Vegetable stock (1 1 and a half cup)

- Half-fat crème fraiche (1 rounded tablespoon)

- Lemon zest (½ lemon)

- Puy lentils (100 grams)

- Smoked haddock fillets (4 Oz)

- Baby spinach leaves (2 Oz)

- Onion (1 small piece, finely chopped)

Directions:

1. Add the lentils, onion, carrot, and celery to a pan over a medium heat.
2. Pour in the stock and then boil for a minute.
3. Stir the vegetables, then lower the heat and let it simmer for 20 minutes.
4. In a separate pan, mix 1 tablespoon of dill, lemon zest, and crème fraiche, and add some salt and pepper.
5. Then in a shallow dish and lay the fish on it. Splash with some water and cover the fish with cling film.
6. Microwave the fish for 4 minutes on medium mode.
7. In the lentil stock, add the spinach, and then add the crème fraiche bowl.
8. Pour the stock into two warmed plates. Place the fish on top of each plate.

9. Top with half tbsp. of dill and serve.

Creamy Cucumber Dill Salad

Ingredients:

- 3 tablespoons rice vinegar

- 1 tablespoon Dijon mustard

- 1 tablespoon honey

- Salt and pepper to taste

- 1 ½ English cucumbers, sliced thin

- 1 small red onion, sliced thin

- 3 tablespoons fresh chopped dill

Directions:

1. Combine the cucumber, red onion and fresh dill in a salad bowl.

2. Whisk together the remaining Ingredients: until smooth.

3. Toss the salad with the dressing and chill until ready to serve.

Easy Mushroom Onion Bisque

Ingredients:

- 4 cups chicken broth or vegetable broth

- 2 tablespoons grass-fed butter

- 1 lbs. sliced mushrooms

- ½ cup whole milk

- Salt and pepper to taste

- 2 tablespoons olive oil

- 3 lbs. Vidalia onions, sliced thin

- 1 teaspoon minced garlic

Directions:

1. Heat the oil in a stockpot over medium heat.

2. Add the onions and cook for 10 minutes until very tender and browned.

3. Stir in the garlic and cook 1 minute then whisk in the broth and bring to a boil.

4. Reduce heat and simmer, covered, for 10 minutes.

5. Remove from heat and puree the soup using an immersion blender.

6. Melt the butter in a skillet over medium-high heat and add the mushrooms.

7. Cook for 10 minutes until browned then season with salt and pepper to taste.

8. Stir the mushrooms and milk into the stockpot and serve the soup hot.

Grilled Salmon Salad

Ingredients:

- 1 lbs. boneless skinless salmon fillet

- Olive oil, as needed

- Salt and pepper to taste

- 6 to 8 cups fresh spring greens

Directions:

1. Preheat the grill to high heat and brush the grates with olive oil.

2. Brush the salmon with olive oil and season with salt and pepper to taste.

3. Place the salmon on the grill and cook for 5 minutes on each side or until just opaque and cooked-through.

4. Divide the spring greens among four salad plates and top with slices of salmon.

5. Serve the salads with your favorite dressing.

Glazed Pork Tenderloin

Ingredients:

- 2 tablespoons coconut oil, additional virgin olive oil, or butter

- ¼ cup beef puree

- 1 tablespoon balsamic vinegar

- 2 tablespoons Dijon mustard

- 1 pound pork tenderloin

- 1 teaspoon ground cardamom

- ½ teaspoon ground dark pepper

- ¼ teaspoon ocean salt

Directions:

1. Preheat the oven to 350°F.

2. On a work surface, rub the tenderloin uniformly with the cardamom, pepper, and salt.

3. In a heatproof heating pan or oven proof skillet over medium-high warmth, warm the oil.

4. Cook the tenderloin, turning at times, for 8 minutes, or until sautéed on all sides.

5. Place in the oven. Cook for 20 minutes, or until a thermometer embedded in the middle registers 160°F and the juices run clear.

6. Expel from the oven and exchange the pork to a cutting board. Let stand for 10 minutes.

7. Place the skillet over medium-high warmth. Include the beef puree and vinegar. Heat to the point of boiling, mixing to uproot any cooked bits.

8. Cook until the mixture is decreased by about half. Rush in the mustard.

9. Cut the pork and shower with the sauce.

Beaded Pork Chops

Ingredients:

- 1 vast egg

- 1 teaspoon sans gluten soy sauce

- ½ cup ground pecans

- 4 boneless pork loin slashes, ¾" thick

- 2 tablespoons olive or coconut oil

- 2 tablespoons ground brilliant flaxseeds

- ½ teaspoon ocean salt

- ½ teaspoon smoked paprika

Directions:

1. On a plate, join the flaxseeds, salt, and paprika.

134

2. In a wide shallow dish, whisk the egg and soy sauce.

3. Place the pecans on a plate.

4. Dunk every hack into the flax mixture, then in the egg mixture, and after that into the pecans to coat.

5. In a huge skillet over medium-high warmth, warm the oil.

6. Cook the pork hacks for 8 minutes, turning once, or until a thermometer embedded sideways in a cleave registers 160°F and the juices run clear.

Slow Cooker French Coq Av Vin

Ingredients:

- 1½ teaspoons herbes de Provence

- 1½ teaspoons ocean salt

- 1½ teaspoons ground dark pepper

- 3 pounds boneless, skinless chicken thighs

- ½ pound solidified pearl onions, defrosted

- ½ cup tomato glue

- 2 tablespoons coconut flour

- 1 cup dry red wine or chicken soup

- 8 ounces button mushrooms

- 6 cuts bacon, coarsely hacked

- 2 huge cloves garlic, minced

Directions:

1. Coat a 5to 6-quart moderate cooker with cooking splash. In the pot, whisk the tomato glue with the coconut flour until the flour breaks down.

2. Whisk in the wine or soup, herbs, salt, and pepper until smooth. Include the chicken, onions, mushrooms, bacon, and garlic.

3. Mix to coat the chicken with the sauce.

4. Cover and cook on high for 2½ to 3 hours or on low for 5 to 6.

Crepes With Ricotta And Strawberries

Ingredients:

Filling

- 1 teaspoon lemon peel

- 2 cups strawberries, halved

- 1 cup ricotta

- 1 teaspoon xylitol or 1 drop liquid stevia or to desired sweetness

Crepes

- ¼ teaspoon sea salt

- 1½ cups almond or carton-variety coconut milk

- 4 eggs

- ¼ cup coconut flour

- ¼ cup golden flaxseed meal

- ¼ teaspoon vanilla extract

Directions:

To prepare the filling:

1. In a small bowl, mix the ricotta, Xylitol or stevia, and lemon peel and then set aside for later use.

To cook the crepes:

2. In a large bowl, mix the coconut flour, flaxseed meal, and salt. In a modest bowl, whisk together the milk, eggs, and vanilla. Now, add the egg mixture to the flour mixture and stir until combined.

3. Coat a small non-stick frying pan with oil and heat over medium high temperature. Measure ⅓ cup of the Batter and pour into the pan, swirling the batter around so it coats the underside of the pan. Cook for 3 minutes, or until the tip of the crepe looks dry. Move

around the crepe and cook for 1 min, or until the bottom is dry. Repetition with the remaining batter, stacking the Crepes as they are prepared.

4. Top each crepe with 2 tablespoons of the ricotta filling and ¼ cup of the strawberries.

Basic Pie Crust

Ingredients:

- 2 teaspoons baking powder

- ½ teaspoon guar gum

- ½ teaspoon xanthan gum

- ½ teaspoon ocean salt

- ½ cup unsalted butter, cut into 3D squares

- 1 egg

- 1 cup walnuts

- 1 cup almond flour, separated

- ⅔ cup ground brilliant flaxseeds

- 1 tablespoon vinegar

- 1 tablespoon water

Directions:

1. In nourishment processor, beat the walnuts until slashed. Include ⅓ cup almond flour, the flaxseeds, baking powder, guar gum, xanthan gum, and salt.

2. Beat until all around mixed. Include the butter and heartbeat 10 times.

3. Include the egg, vinegar, and water, and heartbeat until just consolidated. The mixture will be wet.

4. Dust a work surface and your hands with some almond dinner/flour.

5. Place the mixture on the work surface.

6. Massage the remaining almond supper into the mixture.

7. Structure into a plate. Wrap the mixture with plastic wrap. Refrigerate for no less than 60 minutes.

8. To take off, dust a piece of material paper with almond dinner.

9. Place the mixture on the paper and dust with more almond feast.

10. Top with a second piece of paper. With a rolling pin, move to a 10" round.

11. Peel off the top paper. Place a 9" pie plate upside down over the batter and turn the mixture onto the pie plate.

12. Tenderly peel off the material paper. Trim any shade and crease the edges.

13. Chill until prepared to use. To prebake, preheat the oven to 350°F.

14. Heat for 23 minutes, or until the crust is golden brown and no longer moist to touch.

1.